A Rainbow Book

Animal Chronicles

—*An Odyssey*—

John Behrman, M.D.

Rainbow Books, Inc.
F L O R I D A

Library of Congress Cataloging-In-Publication Data

Behrman, John 1928-
Animal chronicles : an odyssey / John Behrman.
p. cm.
ISBN 1-56825-074-6 (alk. paper)
1. Dogs--United States--Anecdotes. 2. Cats--United States--Anecdotes. 3. Pets--United States--Anecdotes. 4. Behrman, John, 1928- 5. Pet owners--United States--Anecdotes. 6. Physicians--United States--Anecdotes. I. Title.

SF426.2 .B446 2002
636.088'7--dc21 2002069669

Animal Chronicles
—An Odyssey—

ISBN 1-56825-074-6

Published by Rainbow Books, Inc.
P. O. Box 430
Highland City, FL 33846-0430

Editorial Offices and Wholesale/Distributor Orders
Telephone: (863) 648-4420
Email: RBIbooks@aol.com

Individuals' Orders
Toll-free Telephone (800) 431-1579
Online — http://www.allbookstores.com

Cover art from a painting by Joanne Farina

First Printing • Printed in the United States of America.

—Dedication—

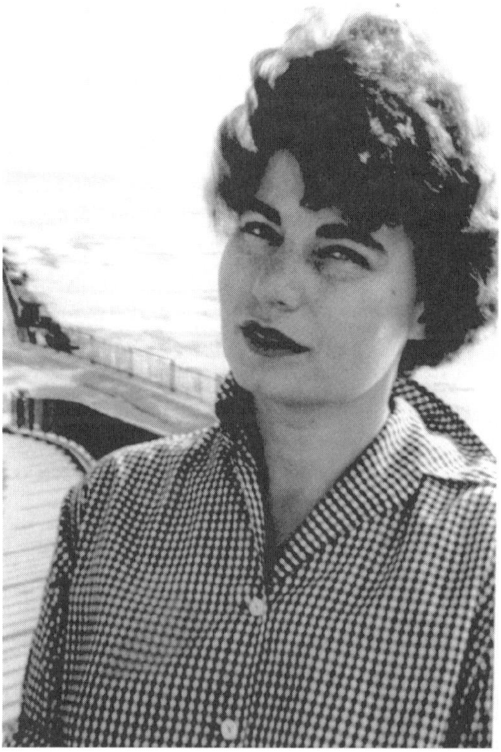

My wife Marilyn passed on in 1995. It was her thought that I write this kind of book, but my loss was so profound that I was unable to be productive for a long time. Marilyn was the joy and marrow of my life and, God willing, I hope to join her when I die.

The Creator must have made trees and vegetation for beauty, animals for innocence and sincerity, and humans to develop technology and make mischief.

Contents

—CHAPTER ONE—

The Spangled Sovereign of Sirius

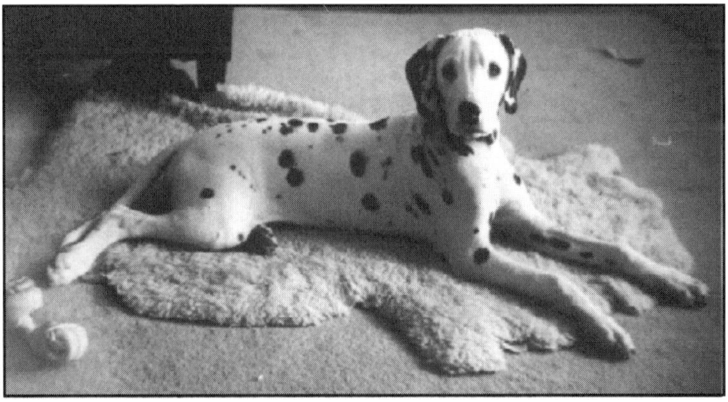

My interest in Dalmatian dogs began while driving my car to an emergency house call at about three o'clock in the morning during the summer of 1963, when I came upon a strikingly beautiful Dalmatian with green eyes, running about in the streets.

Soon after, I went to the library. My curiosity increased after reading about the breed in the American Kennel Club's *The Complete Dog Book*. For good reason, the Dalmatian is sometimes called, "The Firehouse Dog." My wife Marilyn said that she clearly recalled the delight she felt as a small child to see Dalmatians when she passed a firehouse on walks with her aunt Fritzie. Marilyn remembered also that when she was a baby she would lie under the kitchen table, hugging Nellie, the family dog. Nellie's happy odor was permanently etched in her mind.

The only pet I had in my childhood was a salamander that I found and caught one summer at camp. I returned it to its lake on the day my parents came to take me home. Come to think of it, I had a dog for a few hours. One night my father brought home a Spitz puppy. We locked it in the bathroom, and it cried until morning. My mother flatly refused to keep the dog, saying that it would be too much work to take care of an animal. So my father took the dog away and gave it to one of my cousins. I was extremely unhappy, but I had no say in the matter, even though I pleaded every way I could.

On a balmy Saturday afternoon in December of 1963, I was browsing the stores for audio equipment. After losing track of time, as is my wont, I remembered that Marilyn's parents were coming over for dinner. Although I arrived home late, the meal was a great success. Marilyn's mother Jean mentioned that there was an ad in the newspaper for Dalmatian puppies. The next day we thought we had found the ad in the Sunday *New York Times*, and we were off to Oyster Bay, Long Island. On the way to the kennel, Marilyn cautioned more than once that we were only looking, should keep an open mind, and shouldn't feel obliged to immediately adopt a dog. However, for her it was love at first sight of one of the male puppies. She joyfully blurted that he walked like a sailor, and this apparently endeared him to her. I wondered what relevance this might have had to my tour of active duty in the Navy.

Mr. Ruddy, the kennel owner, told us that the puppy we wanted had a serious eye infection, unresponsive to treatment with antibiotic eye drops, and that he had scheduled him for corrective eyelid surgery. If the procedure proved unsuccessful, the puppy was to be put down. This made us intent to rescue him. As we were leaving the kennel, his mother looked in our direction to size us up and bid her son an affectionate goodbye. When I started the car, King (as the puppy was now called) barfed on Marilyn's lap. For sure, I thought, this would bother her, but she just smiled and said that he was upset and that it was okay.

We drove to Marilyn's parents' home, where King received a warm welcome. At dinnertime, he was served a can of cat food but refused it, opting instead for the roast beef the family was having. King won out and was given a Henry the Eighth portion of the roast beef, which he wolfed down. Marilyn's father Milton remarked prophetically that the dog was really something.

When I took King on his first walk, he tripped me, and I fell. He was a quick study, though, and never did it again.

Incidentally, the ad that Jean had brought to our attention appeared in her local newspaper, not in the *New York Times*. This communication snafu was to prove as fortunate as it was fortuitous. Over time, Marilyn and I came to realize that King expanded our horizons and had a positive influence on the course of our life.

In accordance with convention, we took King to a veterinarian for an evaluation of his health. After the examination, the vet opined to our great surprise that the puppy should be put to sleep, because he was not in perfect condition. We flatly rejected his radical solution. King's conjunctivitis was cured with orally administered antibiotics. However, his permanent teeth were tinted yellow by the tetracycline he received. At that time, this side effect was not listed in the product labeling.

Marilyn wore thongs on her feet as she went about the house. She experienced considerable pain from the trauma King inflicted by playfully biting her toes. When she finally came to the end of her rope, he must have had a sixth sense, because, at that point, King abruptly stopped doing it.

King was an irrepressible, good-natured, mischievous bundle of joy. For the fun of it, he became a smiling pickpocket and kleptomaniac. King's appearance and antics brightened the days of almost everyone he met. When a preschool girl saw him for the first time she turned to her mother and excitedly exclaimed, "Circus — circus!"

Birds liked to land on King's back. When King confronted cats, even small ones, they stood their ground. Cattle in an open field didn't take him seriously, either. When he tried to run them, the cattle just looked at him. King always brought broad smiles to the faces of attendants at the entrance gates of outdoor movies by fully expecting them to give him a food treat, and, after a rainfall, he evoked loud laughter from students on the college campus by enthusiastically wallowing in a muddy puddle.

Aunt Fritzie once remarked that King did things naturally that other dogs had to be trained to do for Hollywood films. For a period of time, I frequently worked after office hours in a biochemistry research lab. As I was about to depart for the lab one evening, King began to limp. Marilyn became concerned that something was wrong. I told her that it was a ploy to keep me home. My quick diagnosis proved correct.

In some ways King's psyche was more human than dog. Knowing how to swim is supposedly inherent in canines, but Marilyn had to teach King to swim. For this favor he expressed unrestrained gratitude.

When King was just a few months old we often took him to a park inhabited by numerous squirrels. When he chased one, it invariably ran behind a tree and seemed to disappear. This had the puppy really stumped. One day he had a thinking breakthrough and figured out that the squirrels were climbing up the tree trunks as soon as they were out of sight.

Year after year, King enjoyed watching through a window as kids came to the door for their Halloween treats. He overreacted only once — the time he saw a child in a *Jaws* costume. I think it was the oversized, jagged teeth that captured King's imagination.

In his lifetime, King had several close brushes with death, but dying before his time was not to be his destiny:

> While the dog is man's best friend, a leash is the dog's best friend. We plead guilty to the charge that King was off his leash too often. We stopped for gas while traveling on a six-lane highway, and, as usual, King was let off his leash. Something caught his eyes, and he suddenly took off running in the direction of the highway. Over and over, I screamed his name at the top of my lungs. Thank God, he finally stopped and came back. I was shaken to the core and ashamed of my stupidity. Only one time was King hit by a car. It happened in the parking lot of a motel, and he didn't evidence any signs of injury.
>
> Another time we were riding in our convertible, and King was on his leash. In a state of excitement, he leaped out of the car and was almost dragged to his death.

It was a scorcher in the middle of the summer. During office hours, we left King in the car with the windows partially open. Later, we found him motionless and lying on his back with his legs stretched into the air. We prayed that he was unconscious and not dead. I carried him inside and into the cool of the air conditioning. We applied copious cold compresses and ice bags to him. King responded so slowly that for a while it looked like he wasn't going to make it. Finally his eyes opened, and he started to move. King was on the mend!

It was winter, and we were walking alongside a raging river in the woods. Marilyn had taught King to swim the summer before. Exuberantly, King jumped into the turbulent water. As he was carried downstream, he was being pulled toward the center of the river. We yelled encouragements to him, and with supreme effort he managed to swim to the river bank. We turned the car heater up to maximum and wrapped him in blankets.

There was a foal in a pasture enclosed by a

split rail fence. King decided to investigate. As soon as he went through the fence, the mare, who was quite a distance away, began galloping toward him, intent on protecting her foal. King was unaware that he was in danger of being kicked to death, so it wasn't easy for us to persuade him to come out of the enclosure. Finally he did — but with only a moment to spare!

We were staying at a hotel in the mountains. Our room with a balcony was on the third floor. We never expected King to step off the balcony onto the pitched roof over the room below ours. But he did. He couldn't keep his balance upon landing and slid down to the roof edge, where he fell off. We could hardly believe that he survived a two-story fall without serious injury. Our only explanation for this feat was that King must have been in a state of complete relaxation.

I brought a large state-of-the-art dog house. Its purpose was to give King a place to relax in the backyard, but he misunderstood and rejected it out of hand. To evidence his disdain, he urinated on it. King not only lived in our home, he slept with us on our bed. Obviously, he was taking no chances!

While chatting with a neighbor, the neighbor disclosed that he never saw anything like the way King greeted me on my homecomings. I never gave it a second thought that King was able to easefully jump up and land gently in my open arms.

King seemed to have a special trust in us. Once, he returned from a forest frolic but wouldn't look at us. Forced inspection of his face revealed several porcupine quills stuck in his muzzle. King patiently let me cut the barbs off the quills and pull them out one by one.

Unfortunately, King developed a breast tumor. Although it was benign, it was constantly irritated from being bumped or scraped by the dog's activities. It's amazing that, without being muzzled or restrained in any way, King let me excise it surgically. He didn't wince when the local anesthetic was infiltrated into the surrounding tissues. He lay quietly during the procedure and the suturing of the incision. This was more than an example of blind trust. He had a real understanding that I was removing something causing him considerable annoyance.

Sight unseen, we rented a house from an Army

colonel when we moved to Washington State. Milton, Marilyn's dad, didn't think this was prudent. The house was miles out of town on a dirt road in the boondocks.

The first night, as we were falling asleep, we heard strange noises coming from the utility room. It was the shower wall vibrating as pack rats dropped into the stall. There was a platform on the back porch where they kept their treasures, many shiny objects and other acquisitions. We tried to get rid of the rats every way we could think of. We sealed all cracks and small openings. We set traps, and the rats ate the bait without springing the trap mechanisms. We put out d-CON (bait poisoned with anticoagulant). The rats ate the d-CON, and to pay for the treat, they left several of their prized possessions. Bartering is one of the things pack rats are famous for. That's why they are also called trade rats. After the first time, they wouldn't eat the d-CON again. This display of intelligence should not be underestimated.

During the daytime, the rats were away somewhere. They returned every evening at dusk and spent most of their time in the walls of the house, making threatening, scratching noises. In the middle of the night, as they ran back and forth on the top of our roof, King growled. He didn't know how to get rid of them, either. In the end, the rats won, and we moved.

King's originality was all but boundless. One of his hobbies was to completely denude the fuzz from tennis balls, until they became just plain rubber balls.

Instead of seeking shade on the hottest summer days, King would lie out in the open. I remarked that only "mad dogs and Englishmen" sought out the blazing midday sun. Imagine how hot his black spots became as they absorbed the sun's rays in contrast to how cool the areas of his white coat felt around the spots.

At the age of twelve, King's back leg muscles began to atrophy and his bark became thready. He had a fatal neurologic illness. Marilyn nursed him to the end, saying she would never put a dog of ours down, because it would be a break in trust, and the dog would know what was being done.

King was almost fourteen years old, when Marilyn and I were at the circus in Manhattan and I received a "telepathic message from King" to come home immediately. We got back as fast as we could to find King completely paralyzed. I placed him on a couch, and we were with him as he died. Then a most miraculous thing happened . . .

King was essentially dead, lying on his side. For about four minutes, all of his paralyzed legs moved in a magnificent rhythmic gait, as though he were proudly entering heaven and being received by God and an abundance of cheering angels . . .

When King's legs ceased to run, I buried his body in our backyard.

—Chapter Two—

Sybil

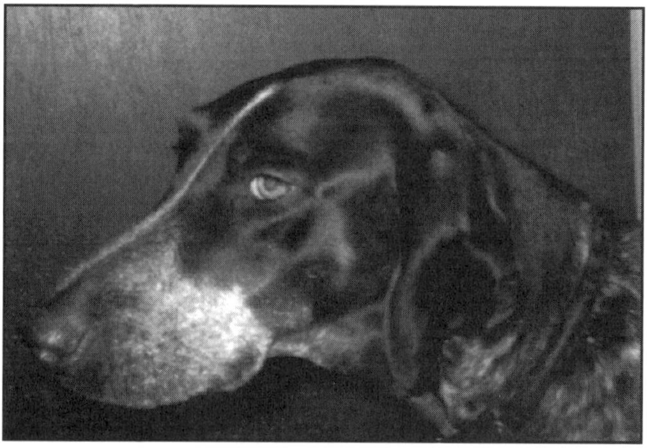

In the summer of 1965, we moved to Norman, Oklahoma, where I had taken a position on the Student Health Service of the University of Oklahoma and was given the opportunity to pursue my enzyme research as a principal investigator at the medical school.

Nine days before the fall semester began, Marilyn, King and I took an automobile tour through New

Mexico and Texas. My pocket clock was ruined by swimming in a Holiday Inn pool with the clock in the pocket of my swim trunks. I replaced it with a pocket watch. Because I was hesitant, the proprietor of the shop guaranteed to take the watch back, no questions asked, during the first year. It was an offer I couldn't refuse. I grew sentimental about that watch, which still keeps perfect time thirty-six years later.

In El Paso, we gave King Mexican food for the first time. It became his favorite food ever after.

On the interstate between Santa Fe and Albuquerque, we had a flat tire. As hard as I tried, I couldn't remove the wheel to put the spare on. That night we slept in the car on the shoulder of the highway. Early the next morning, a trucker stopped to help us and removed the wheel without difficulty, explaining that the threads were reversed on my Pontiac Bonneville. The night before, I was actually tightening the lug nuts in my effort to loosen them.

During the 1965 Christmas season, we vacationed in Texas at South Padre Island and some border towns. In the late afternoon, after checking into a five-star motel, we went for a walk on the impressive grounds. A friendly, young, female German Shorthaired Pointer suddenly appeared. She had no ID on her collar, was quite thin and seemed to be on her own. She looked super, and I remarked that her owner was very lucky. As I stroked her, I felt several tumors on her back.

On the following days, she would appear whenever we walked the grounds. One evening, we brought King some food from a Mexican restaurant. Drawn by the aroma, the German Shorthair followed us into our room. King stood back as she devoured his favorite food. When we were loading our luggage into the car to go home, the German Shorthair appeared. I wanted to take her with us.

We were about to drive off, and Marilyn said, "Open a back door and let it be her choice."

Sybil thought about it for a while, and we anxiously waited to see what she would do. She decided to join us and entered the car on her own. That night, she slept on the floor in our family room. In the morning, her tumors were gone — because they weren't tumors at all. Several giant ticks had abandoned her coat and were positioned on the carpet. This must have been the first time in a long while that Sybil slept indoors.

Sybil was a hunter par excellence. The north campus of Oklahoma University consisted of open fields providing a natural habitat for a variety of small wild animals. Sybil's brain contained a computer that automatically set her off on the optimum trajectory to intercept rabbits fleeing for their lives. King could barely keep up with her lightning speed, because he had put on some extra pounds before Sybil's arrival. He trimmed down rapidly under her tutelage.

Occasionally, Sybil ranged far out of our call and sight. We would comb the streets and roads by car and most of the time we would find her. On occasion, she would be lost and we had to go home with only one dog. Once, our postman brought her back after she was gone several days. She was heat beat and dehydrated. We should have kept her leashed more consistently, but knowing her natural inclinations, we didn't want her to feel like a prisoner.

The following vignettes capture the essence of sweet Sybil:

> I came home for lunch and Marilyn and a neighbor were in the neighbor's backyard looking for Sybil, who to them seemed to have vanished into thin air. The gate on the fence around the yard was closed. I surveyed the scene and noted that the door to a small room on the back of the house was ajar. I directed my voice

at the door and loudly called, "Come on out Sybil. I know you're in there." Sybil, who was hiding in the room, pranced out. She was delighted that I appreciated her high jinks. Sybil always had a precious sense of humor.

We were on our way to a medical meeting in Phoenix. Before we left, Marilyn had prepared a dozen hard-boiled eggs that she had purchased at her favorite egg farm. She placed the unshelled eggs in a cooler, which she placed behind her seat. During the trip, Sybil stayed on the back seat. When we were ready for our snack, Marilyn pulled the cooler up front, and, to our amazement, it was empty. Since we hadn't heard any crunching of eggshells, we concluded that Sybil feasted on all twelve of the eggs, she took each one in her mouth and chewed it silently with her lips closed so as to avoid detection.

King tended to be a juvenile delinquent. He often had a defiant attitude and to get attention endlessly thought up doggy pranks. Sybil eventually became his personal police dog and reprimanded him by barking whenever she caught him in the act. We found that this amusing behavior was quite useful.

One night, on our way back from the South campus, where the dogs customarily took their last run for the day, we smelled a strong obnoxious odor in our car. We thought that the nearby sewage treatment plant had exploded. But when we entered our house, the odor followed us in. The dogs had been sprayed by a skunk. Incidentally, tomato juice doesn't remove skunk aroma.

Sybil wouldn't stop eating mice. It was probably key to her survival in Texas. We used to watch her gulp them down. I started to carry an emetic with me. Within three minutes of administering the injection, she vomited up the four mice she swallowed. We hoped this maneuver would help discourage her from dining on mice.

It didn't rain often in Norman, but when it did, it was frequently torrential. Sybil could forecast a downpour forty-eight hours in advance. She did this by pointing her nose to the sky in the direction the storm would be coming from. King could predict cloudbursts twenty-four hours beforehand. Once, he barked at the sky and the gully washer that followed was hurricanesque.

While attending a professional meeting in Chicago, we let the dogs run about one evening in Montrose park along Lake Michigan. When I was in medical school, we had lived close by. Before we could stop her, Sybil caught and ate a sick bird. The bird must have been poisoned because Sybil became very sick for several days. She never fully recovered from this episode. She began to waste away, but we didn't see it, perhaps because we loved her so much.

Sybil died on Marilyn's birthday, February 18, 1968. In retrospect, we saw the progressive weight loss in her photographs. Postmortem examination performed by the peerless veterinarian, Dr. J. G. Hemphill disclosed that her kidneys had no functioning tissue left. Probably another factor affecting her renal function was her habit of drinking lawn runoffs that contained toxic chemicals. She may have been getting a high from the lawn chemicals. Also, mouse viruses are known to attack the kidney. I wonder if eating mice that carry virus explains why so many cats die in kidney failure.

I buried Sybil's body in our backyard. When I patted down the grave with the shovel, King growled at me.

—CHAPTER THREE—

The Racy Rani of Rainier

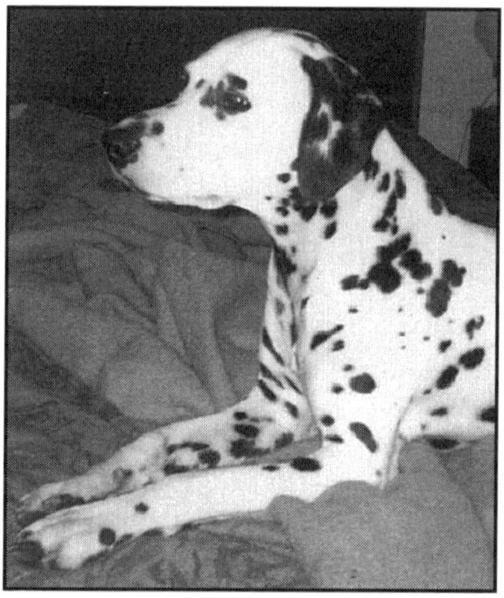

In June of 1968, I was appointed director of the student health center at Washington State College, which subsequently became Central Washington State University. We spent the summer at the beach with Marilyn's parents, and I practiced as a *locum tenens* for a Manhattan physician.

At the end of the summer, we traveled at high

speeds on our journey to the left coast. Crossing Montana, we cruised at ninety miles an hour. Marilyn drove the Oldsmobile and I the Pontiac. At each gas stop, King switched cars. On the day after our arrival as we drove about town, we heard a jingling sound coming from one of the wheels on the Olds. On removal of the hubcap, we found three of the five lugs completely off their bolts. Our trip had almost ended in tragedy.

Mrs. Messner, the wife of one of the partners in the principal medical group in Ellensburg, had Dalmatian puppies for sale. Life with Sybil made it clear that two dogs in the family was the way to go. Marilyn inquired and was told that only one puppy was not spoken for. It was the smallest one in the litter. Marilyn purchased her on the spot.

We were still living in the Colonel's house with the rats, and because Rani liked to explore every nook and cranny, I feared for her safety. Just before a real estate agent was to show us a rental house, we left Rani at the Messner's. We wanted to give the impression that we had only one dog instead of two so that we would appear to be more desirable tenants. I can't forget Rani's forlorn face that clearly said, "Why are you doing this? Don't you love me? What did I do?"

Rani was born on August 1, 1968. She was quite

an innovative dog with a delightful temperament. Rani was also an escape artist, and when confined in a container of some sort could almost always figure her way out. She struck up a friendship with a young Beagle. Whenever he visited, even though she couldn't see him, she knew that he was waiting for her outside the house. They would tirelessly play together for hours.

Rani thought that it was great fun to run the cattle grazing in an enormous field behind our house. She could control the entire herd with no difficulty. One look at her coming toward them, and they were all off in a great stampede. Ranchers shoot dogs that run their cattle because the weight loss cuts down on their profit. Rani found a steer skull that became her pet. If we returned home late at night, she would sit in the field with her favorite skull, frustrating all efforts to get her into the house so we could get to sleep.

I have a pleasant remembrance of Rani's first bark, as she was standing on a couch. She would jump onto our dinner table and help herself. Rani's favorite was baked potato. Those Idaho potatoes were the best we ever had. I think it was because we were so close to Idaho. Have you discovered that Maine lobster tastes better in Maine than anywhere else and that Maryland crab tastes better in Maryland?

In June 1970, we returned to New York city because I had accepted a position in the pharmaceutical industry to design and monitor clinical research studies. When we arrived after dark in Belle Harbor, we decided to give the dogs a needed run on the beach before proceeding to Marilyn's parents' home. Rani had never seen an ocean and ran along the shoreline. We were dismayed as she distanced out of sight. As a small child, I became disoriented at the beach and couldn't find my way home. While Marilyn continued the search, I went back to our automobile which was parked three blocks in from the water. Rani was sitting on the hood of the car waiting for us. In about half an hour, Marilyn returned. She was astonished that Rani hadn't lost her bearings.

We settled into an apartment on the thirtieth floor at Sixty-sixth Street and Central Park West. It was within walking distance of my office in the General Motors building. On a warm Saturday afternoon in October 1970, we were in Central Park with the dogs when Rani became distressed. We had been unaware that she was pregnant but took her straight home. She jumped on our bed and in a few minutes began giving birth to five completely white puppies. Their spots began to appear after about ten days.

Marilyn named the two males Bigboy and Sweetheart and the three females Onedot, Threedot and Pepper. Naturally, Rani doted on them and King just tolerated them with curiosity. Four of the five puppies were sold to young couples residing in New Jersey. Each puppy left by the order of its spots in that the most heavily spotted went first and so on. Bigboy had the fewest spots, and his story will be told in the next chapter.

City life didn't agree with Rani, who, from the get-go, was used to roaming the open country. She was a free spirit. One day, while running great circles in Central Park, she took off on a tangent and began covering ground rapidly. Marilyn went after her questioning people along the way as to whether they saw a Dalmatian running free. Most of them said that they had and they indicated the direction she was going. I went back to the apartment building and waited at the service entrance on Sixty-fifth Street. This was the exit we had to use when the dogs were with us because they weren't allowed in the lobby. After what seemed to be a very long time, Rani ambled down the street from the direction of the park. I again marveled at her sense of direction. Marilyn said that Rani had practically covered the entire park on her escapade.

On Thanksgiving Eve in 1971, we moved to New Jersey. Overriding consideration in our choice of the home was that there was almost an acre of land behind the house. We had a six-foot stockade fence built so that King, Rani and Bigboy could roam around in relative safety, and Marilyn was spared the wear and tear of walking them on leashes. Just behind the house was a lawn area, and the rest of the property was a wooded forest. Rani was happy again. Occasionally, she would howl more melodiously than a wolf and Bigboy would join in, but he never howled on his own. Rani enjoyed robust health and seemed to be a superdog. She spent a lot of time playfighting with Bigboy, teaching him several dirty tricks. After a heavy snowstorm, she didn't hesitate to run out of the house, cutting a path for the other dogs through snow that was as high as she was tall.

In this world, nothing good lasts for very long. In 1975, Rani developed heartworm infection and had difficulty breathing even at rest. She was cured by a course of medication. Until then, we thought heartworm was common only in southern states where mosquitos are more prevalent. Ever since, we give the dogs preventive medicine every month. One day in 1978, Rani had a major convulsion. I thought something had lodged in her throat and put my fingers way back to pull it out. Nothing was there, but the nerve reflex it generated stopped her convulsions. From that point, it was downhill all the way. We consulted several vets, and none could figure out what was wrong with her. A year later, she died during the night on the floor at the foot of our bed.

I buried Rani's body next to King's grave in our backyard.

—CHAPTER FOUR—

Noble Prince Bigboy

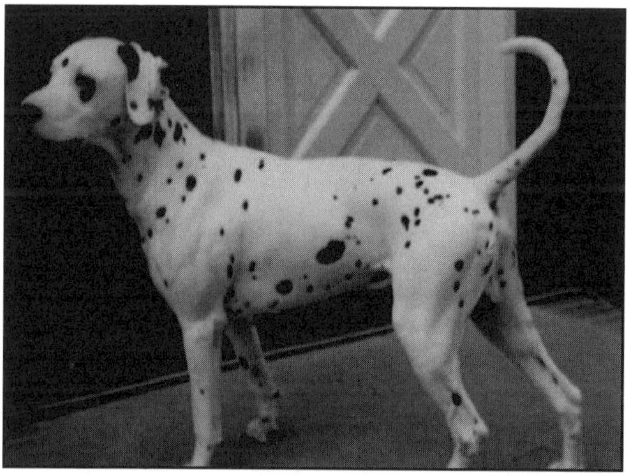

At the very outset, Bigboy differed from his littermates. He was stronger, larger and silkier. Like his father before him, he had a Dudley nose. Also, his behavior was distinctive. Wanting not to be confined to their enclosure at bedtime, the other puppies ran and hid as best they could. Bigboy went to the enclosure and pawed it to tell us that he was ready to be placed inside for the night.

When potential buyers arrived, Bigboy tried hard to be chosen, but he never was. Perhaps it was because of his homely face and the paucity of his spots. After the first two or three puppies were adopted, he seemed to lose interest in being selected. I wondered if he wanted to avoid being disappointed again or if he was beginning to relate to us. Even after his brother and sisters were sold, those who came to look at him decided they weren't interested. Finally, in response to our ad, a man called and said that he wanted to use him as an overnight guard dog in his liquor store in the roughest section of the city. That was the last straw. Marilyn, already attached to Bigboy, wouldn't hear of it. As much as she was against taking on a third dog, she decided that Bigboy would stay.

We took Bigboy to the vet for his first examination and shots. The puppy didn't relate to him. As we left the office, the vet said, "If you want my advice, take him out to a field somewhere and shoot him."

During his first thirteen months, Bigs lived on Central Park West in New York City. Here are some anecdotes from that portion of his life:

In my absence, a floor-repair worker tried to come on to Marilyn, and she felt threatened.

Bigboy was only three months old, but, by growling, Bigs appeared sufficiently menacing to turn the man off. In fact, the man acted as though he couldn't get out of the apartment fast enough. On his own, Bigboy had sized up the situation correctly. There had been no prompting from Marilyn.

In Central Park, Bigboy's two favorite pastimes were chasing horses that people were riding and breaking up flocks of pigeons in the sheep meadow.

My parents were over for dinner, and Bigs was only two months old. He stood in front of my mother and barked for several minutes. His behavior was inexplicable. Although he wasn't admonished, Bigs never again barked at another human being.

Marilyn's sister Gail visited with her two small daughters. The dogs were milling about when our guests were at the door, preparing to leave. Each girl received a harmless nip on the buttocks. All thought Rani was guilty because

Bigboy moved so fast he escaped detection. Was Bigs attracted to them and expressing affection? He never again bit another being.

When we rode in one of the building elevators, and it stopped on a floor to admit passengers, King and Bigboy became terrors. They put on an Academy Award performance of ferocity that included climbing the elevator walls. The only tenant they liked was B. B. King, whom they welcomed aboard. When an occupied elevator stopped on our floor, we didn't dare enter. We patiently waited for an empty one to arrive.

Until it became to large, Rani used to hold Bigboy's head in her mouth. He didn't like it at all but couldn't do anything about it. When he was older, he could have done the same to her but didn't.

For two weeks in the summer of 1970, we rented a vacation house in a remote region of upstate New York. While Rani and King were permitted to roam, Bigboy wasn't. One day, we tried him off the leash. Like his parents, he wandered off exploring but, unlike them, he didn't return. I set out on a search and, with a stroke of great luck, finally found him about two hundred feet away from me in the woods, looking worried and nonplused. He could hear my voice but couldn't tell the direction it was coming from. He stood motionless as I walked right up to him. Too bad he didn't inherit his mother's extraordinary sense of direction.

Just after the movers had emptied the apartment of our things on the day we were relocating to New Jersey, Marilyn stepped out of the apartment with the dogs. They were in a merry mood and exuberantly ran forty feet down the hall to the elevator. Marilyn was toppled over onto the carpet and, as she held fast to the leashes, was rapidly dragged in the prone position all the way to the elevator.

I very much wanted the stockade fence to be in place before we moved to our new home. Accordingly, I scheduled its construction well in advance. However, the fence builder proved unreliable and didn't get around to doing the job until three weeks after we took up residence. On completion of the fence, he came inside to receive payment. At that point, Bigs did something truly unusual. He quietly took one of the man's sleeves into his mouth and, silently holding on, walked with him for the entire time he was in the house. Bigs finally let go of his sleeve when he departed.

We thought it would be beneficial to give Bigboy obedience lessons. On his first visit, the professional trainer went to work with him in the backyard. No matter what techniques the trainer tried, Bigs just glued his eyes on the trainer and ran circles around him. As he left, the trainer said, "I won't be back." We asked why, and he told us that he was afraid for his life.

I let Bigboy and Rani out the back door, and Rani took off after a squirrel on the lawn. Bigs followed in close pursuit and easily overtook her. He caught and killed the squirrel. After that, Bigboy never again killed or even hunted another animal.

Frazzle was a large male Collie who lived in the house directly across the street. Bigs ran over and grasped him by the neck. Frazzle put up absolutely no resistance, and Bigboy responded by releasing him without harm.

There was a giant turtle in the woods behind our house. Bigs would often find it and, for the fun of it, pick it up and run with it. Bigs never applied enough jaw pressure to injure the turtle.

Bigs came upon a snake and watched it for a while. Later, he communicated his discovery to us by crawling along on his belly.

One night, just before we went to sleep, Marilyn went downstairs to get something in the foyer. She turned right around and came back to the bedroom where Bigboy was listening suspiciously to her every footstep, as though he wasn't sure of who was on the stairs. As Marilyn entered the bedroom, he sniffed her scent to make positive identification. Bigs may have been somewhat paranoid, but we couldn't have hoped to have had more foolproof protection.

When friends, relatives or other guests visited, Bigboy was a perfect gentleman, but he never tried to make points with anyone. Occasionally, a stranger on the street would ask permission to pet him. Prudently, we always declined. Like most dogs, Bigs was intensely devoted to his family. There just wasn't room in his heart for anyone else.

The only treat Bigboy relished more than ice cream was ice cream topped with whipped cream. For convenience, we dispensed the whipped cream from aerosol cans. I think that the propellant may have been a casual factor in the development of urinary tract stones that made him unable to void. The vet took x-rays but overlooked the small white spots on the films. His diagnosis was urate stones. More than ninety percent of urinary tract calculi in Dalmatians consists of urates.

I looked at the x-rays and thought that the stones weren't urate because they weren't radiolucent. Bigs almost bled to death during the operation. A posterior urethrostomy was fashioned so that the flow of urine was diverted before reaching Bigboy's penis. He then urinated through a surgically constructed proximal stoma. Three months later, the opening spontaneously closed and his urination returned to normal. Without whipped cream, Bigs didn't get any more calcium stones.

Bigboy repeatedly contracted ear infections. We tried several antibiotic ear drops without success. Our postman suggested using baking soda, which cleared his infection and two subsequent ones. But then it failed to work on a particularly severe infection. After pondering what to do, Marilyn came up with the thought that it might be a fungus infection, and she was right. We instilled antifungal medication into his ears and the infection went away.

As Bigboy matured, his father became determined to expel him and harassed him mercilessly. You probably know that this is not an uncommon occurrence when male dogs live together, especially if a female dog is also present. Bigs loved King very much, and, although he had become larger and stronger than his father, he put up no defense when attacked. One evening, Bigs was napping and King, who was about twenty feet away, developed a strange look on his face. We called to Bigs to awaken him. He woke up just in time to seize King's snout. With repeated encouragements from us, Bigs finally abandoned his passivity.

King's next attack came in the backyard. Before that, King hadn't moved against Bigs in the outdoors. The fight was fearsome. Bigs managed to get King by the neck and wouldn't let go. Someone once told us that any dogfight could be stopped with a garden hose. We believed it, but it isn't true. At a distance of a few inches, I directed the full force of the water at Bigboy's head with no effect. Only when King stopped struggling, and conceded defeat, did the battle end.

A final episode occurred one night in our bedroom. This fight was horrendous and King's blood was spattered on the walls. He almost died from his wounds. After that, we consistently kept them apart until King's death three years later.

On Thanksgiving in 1977, Bigboy ate an enormous amount of turkey and, this time, he did form urate stones. Turkey is high in protein purines. The Dalmatian metabolizes purines to uric acid, just as we humans do. All other dog breeds further oxidize uric acid to allantoin. That is why Dalmatian urine doesn't leave white spots on the grass while other dogs' urine does. Twice a day, I was able to pass a catheter into his distended bladder to relieve him. He endured this painful procedure with cooperation and appreciation. We alkalinized his urine with sodium bicarbonate to help dissolve the stones, and he received allopurinol to block the formation of uric acid.

After three weeks, his urine stream returned. Bigs was able to eat most meats without trouble but turkey, liver, sardines, shellfish, eggs and certain other foods are so high in protein purines that they are bad for male Dalmatians. During the remaining eight years of his life, Bigboy had no recurrence of urinary tract stones.

Rani died in 1979 just two years after King's death. Bigboy, who was now the only dog, suffered a major depressive reaction. His grief was so profound, the thought that he might not survive crossed my mind. At least twice a week, we began taking him for long automobile rides in the Watchung Mountains. While Bigs was in the front passenger seat, he became animated. The drives were truly therapeutic, and his mood slowly started to lift. I wondered whether automobiles were important to him in a previous life. During one of our excursions, we caught sight of a Dalmatian in a field. She looked somewhat like Rani. Crossing her path was prognostic because, within a few days, a young female Dal was brought to our home by members of an animal rescue group. Her name was Duchess, and her timely arrival proved salutary for Bigboy.

In August of 1982, we temporarily moved back to Norman Oklahoma. The rat and rat-flea population in the southwest had escalated out of control. The rat flea is the vector for the bacterium *Yersinia pestis*, which caused the plague. In the Middle Ages, Europe's population was devastated by the plague, also known as the Black Death. Just before we returned to New Jersey, Bigboy caught it and had the worst type, the pneumonic form. He could hardly breathe on our trip home. Marilyn kept him alive with high doses of tetracycline and supportive care. It was a close call but he managed to survive. At the time, many New Mexico license plates bore the maxim, "Land of the flea, home of the plague."

Bigboy developed a neurologic illness similar to King's. Marilyn tried alternative therapies. He had intermittent remissions, but his course was progressive. I returned home from my office one night and Marilyn came outside to meet me and said, "It's all over." Two hours before my arrival, Bigs had died while looking into her eyes. As I was kneeling on the floor hugging Bigs and telling him I loved him, his body quaked. It's amazing that he stayed in a state of suspended animation that long waiting to say goodbye to me.

Two days later, as I carried Bigboy's body into the backyard to bury it, Duchess and Coco (Chapter Seven) rejoiced briefly because they thought that going outdoors would revive him.

—Chapter Five—

Duchess

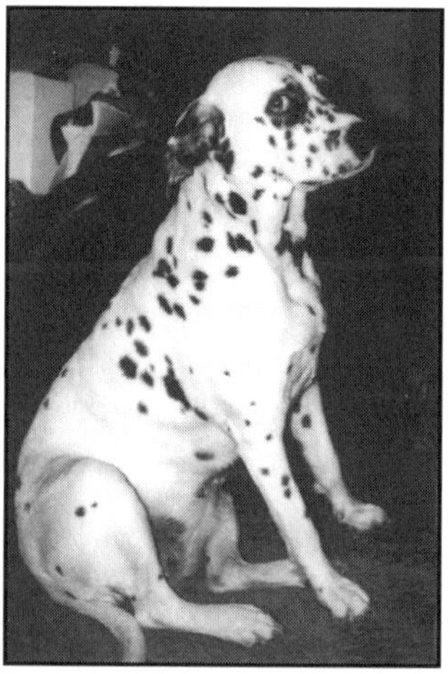

Duchess was three years old when she was brought to us. We were told by the members of the animal rescue team that she had been abused and abandoned.

Ducky was the most laid-back, even-tempered and tractable of all our dogs.

Shortly after she arrived, we had Ducky spayed. On the very day of surgery on the drive home, I had to stop suddenly and she flew off the back seat, bounced off the back of the front seat and landed with a thud on the floor. How lucky it was that she didn't hemorrhage or suffer some other posttraumatic sequela.

Ducky never hunted; however, she did evidence a lot of curiosity about the wild denizens in the yard. I observed her watch a spider creep a long distance across a garden hose. Harming the spider was a thought that would never occur to her.

Ducky emitted the aroma of a fragrant candy.

First thing every morning, Ducky and I had a wrestling match in bed. She was surprisingly strong but I was able to restrain her in either a half nelson or a full nelson. Then I would say, "I've got you now, and I can't let you go." This didn't phase Ducky. She tried to work free of the hold while I held on tight for a good while. Not once did Ducky ever bark or whimper.

Ducky's protective instinct was illustrated by the concern she showed for me as Marilyn gave me haircuts. Ducky must have thought that haircutting was painful. She didn't know for sure because Dalmatians never take haircuts. In fact, except for nail clipping and a bath, no preparation for dog shows is needed.

When Marilyn fed carrots to our Zebronkey (see the next chapter), the dogs were given their share. The others were proactive, but Ducky patiently waited so unobtrusively that Marilyn often failed to notice her. Occasionally, I reminded Marilyn by saying, "The Duck would like to have a piece."

On each dog's birthday, we would throw a party. When it wasn't her birthday, Ducky felt left out and became saddened. We remedied this by singing the "Happy Birthday" song to her as well at the other dog's celebration.

After we returned from our second sojourn in Oklahoma, Marilyn told me that Ducky finally felt secure because we brought her back with us. She had been emotionally scarred by being abandoned by her first owners.

Ducky appeared ancient when she died in 1987. I buried her body in our backyard.

—Chapter Six—

The Zebronkey

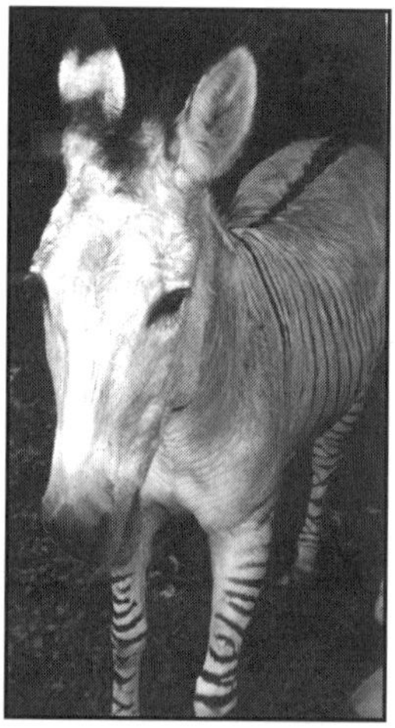

In 1982, my office was located in Oklahoma City. During the initial months, my spare time was taken up with preparations for my specialty board examinations in occupational and preventive medicine. In November, after my studying was out of the way, I toured the Oklahoma City Zoo. The last captive creature that I came to was a Zebronkey, which is a cross between a Zebra and a Donkey. Aside from her stripes, the first attribute that caught my attention were her wide, winsome eyes that reflected serenity, intelligence and self-assurance. I felt a degree of compassion for her. What was a nice girl like her doing in a place like this? I bought some Monkey Chow at the zoo store and, through the bars of her cage, fed it into her soft gentle mouth.

In the ensuing months, I visited the Zebronkey about twice a week. One stormy winter day when I went to the zoo, the lady who sold admission tickets said, "You're crazy to come here in this terrible weather." That afternoon, I was the only visitor on their premises. Marilyn located some treats at a horse emporium where she found out that the Zebronkey was well-known throughout the area. She would pack treats and sugar cubes for me to hand feed to the Zebronkey. My times at the zoo became the high points of my workweek. The Zebronkey had a powerful presence and a genial disposition. As she caught sight of me, she greeted me with a neigh.

In January 1983, as the time to return to New Jersey drew close, I casually mentioned to Marilyn that the only thing I would miss was seeing the Zebronkey. Without hesitation, she asked, "Why don't you take her with you?" The next day, I visited the director of the zoo, Dr. Lawrence Curtis, and said that I wondered whether the Zebronkey could be purchased. To my surprise, he replied, "Yes." The director confided that there were plans to transfer her to a zoo in a northern state.

This didn't augur well for the Zebronkey. Dr. Curtis didn't know how old she was but estimated five years of age. Her previous owner had donated her to the zoo. Searching the Yellow Pages, we found one person, Mr. Carl Paramore, who was willing and able to transport her.

Once back in New Jersey, we began to build a stable in our garage. Our work platform consisted of two tables placed side by side. The tabletops were made of doors that we obtained from the lumber yard that sold us the wood and plans to construct the stable. Because the time we could spend on the project was limited, and because of our inexperience, progress was slow.

When Ze arrived on March 24, 1983, the stable sections were still unfinished. It took two more weeks for completion. In the interim, we had an unusually long stretch of cold, rainy days that put Ze under the weather. Ze had a traveling companion on her journey. It was a racehorse bound for New England.

For a good while, Ze wouldn't debark from the trailer. Marilyn thought of rolling sugar cubes around in her hands. Ze must have perceived Marilyn's scent on them because it did the trick. She went to the center of the yard, stood there and didn't look back. Mr. Paramore surveyed her new habitat and said, "She's going to like it here." As he left, he remarked that, with the Zebronkey, we would always have something to talk about with guests.

At first, Ze was spooked by the dogs, who considered her an intruder on their turf. My primary concern was their safety, so I made an arrangement with a horse farm to take her. When three men came to collect her, she evaded their efforts — but they persisted. Then Ze ran to Marilyn for help, placing her head under Marilyn's arm. At that moment, Marilyn decided that Ze would stay. Eventually, Ze developed a maternal attitude toward the dogs, and they, in turn, became her good friends.

Marilyn chose a perfect site for the stable on the north side where the woods meet the clearing. The stable has no wall or door facing south, so it has a direct view of the house. In winter, Ze gets maximum exposure to the sun and protection from the north wind. At the zoo, one side of her stable was completely open, and we copied this configuration. Ze seemed pleased as she watched us assemble the structure, which measured eight feet by eight feet, with thousands of nails.

Ze quickly made herself at home. She started by eating the wood shingles right off of the house. We repeatedly chased her away, but to no avail. To solve the problem, Marilyn had a split-rail fence erected at a distance of ten feet from the back of the house.

There were bare spots in the clearing. We were filling them in with grass squares and, to our chagrin, as we worked, Ze ate many of them before we could position them on the ground.

Ze became popular with the squirrels, birds, rabbits and raccoons. She is nonthreatening to them and they help themselves to her Horse Chow and hay.

When she was young, Ze let off steam by running. She was heavy-hoofed enough to make our house vibrate and even shake a little.

Ze is half wild and can't be ridden. Being a hybrid, similar to a mule, she can't bear offspring.

During the "bug" months, June to October, Ze used to stand in the flow coming from our home's air conditioning compressor. We improved on this with a powerful shop fan placed in a location convenient for her. When the insects became overwhelming, we applied a repellent, but it didn't work. In fact, it seemed to attract the biting bugs. Next, we tried spraying her with insecticide, but she wouldn't abide an aerosol. She does permit the application of flea-and-tick carpet powder, and, if it doesn't rain, the powder protects her for two to three days. She quickly caught on to this stratagem and now looks forward to having the powder rubbed in.

We always enjoyed meals alfresco. Uninvited, Ze joined in by eating everything in sight, including the napkins. We had to move our table and chairs to our side of the split-rail fence to avoid her disruptive participation. She would come to the fence for handouts, and we obliged by giving her fruits, vegetables, bread and an occasional paper napkin.

Ze snorts to express satisfaction. She no longer whinnied but would kiss Marilyn on the lips. Ze is self-reliant and has routines that occupy many hours and take her to every corner of the wooded area.

Severe storms sometimes fell trees that land on the stockade fence, leaving gaping holes. Rarely, an aberrant wind comes along and blows down a section of fence. Ze never goes through any of these openings.

Having no desire to escape from Utopia, she stays on the property. When workers come to repair the damage, she walks up close to watch them and make sure they're doing a good job.

It became apparent that on very cold nights Ze suffered and needed to have the barn heated. We had electricians suspend infrared lamps from the stable ceiling, which is high enough to leave plenty of clearance for her. We had masons install a concrete floor within which the electricians positioned heating mats as the concrete was being laid. A carpenter insulated the walls with Styrofoam retained by plywood. As weather conditions require, the floor heat and either two or all four of the infrared units can be turned on from inside the house.

Whenever the water hose froze, we would have to carry water a considerable distance from our back door to the stable. This was burdensome and dangerous when ice was on the ground. We had a plumber run a water pipe four feet underground from the house to the stable. At this depth, the water in the pipe stays liquid at subfreezing temperatures. The water flows from a nozzle at the top of an upright extension to the pipe. When the valve is closed, the extension empties because the water it contained drains out of its bottom end at a depth of four feet.

There is an extensive growth of chives all over our property. Ze relishes them. We discovered that always when the chives fall over in the spring, there are no more cold days coming; and when they appear in the fall, there are no more warm days to anticipate.

Ze injured her front left ankle and subsequently injured it twice again. We called a large-animal hospital and two vets came over. They tried to examine Ze, but she wouldn't cooperate. They suggested tranquilizing her using a dart gun. We didn't like the idea. Ze's ankle became fixed in a bent position, and she favors her front left extremity.

In 1991, at the Christmas dinner with the office and nursing staffs, I noticed a large color painting propped up on the floor in front of our table and said that it looked like Ze. The staff was amused and said, "It is Ze." The painting was a super Christmas present. I wondered how the likeness could have been so perfect. They explained that one of them stole Ze's photograph from my desk and loaned it to another, whose artist mother did the splendid portrait. When we showed the painting to Ze, she became very curious. I think she figured out that it was of her.

When Ze was young, we gave her sugar cubes. As she aged, she would limp on the following day. Also when she was young, she enjoyed having beer with us. We never noted any negative effect from the beer but discontinued it when she became elderly. Now, her eyelashes are white, her mane and the wide dark brown stripe running the length of her back are turning gray and there are deep depressions above her eyes.

On July 7, 1998, the township sanitary inspector appeared at the door. He informed me that the health department received complaints of nuisance odors emanating from my property. I invited him to make a survey of the enclosed area. On August 6, 1998, he sent a formal follow-up letter outlining the situation. I responded to his letter with the following comments:

> The Zebronkey has lived here fifteen and a half years without incident or complaint.
>
> You agreed at your on-site inspection that no odor was detectable. Others have confirmed your perception.
>
> The new neighbor who made the complaints resides more than one hundred and fifty feet from Ze's enclosure.

> The potential presence of a nuisance odor should be subjected to unbiased reality testing in the field.

I haven't heard any more from the health department in years.

Marilyn said that one of the best things I ever did was securing Ze. I reminded her that, since it was her idea, she deserved the credit.

My customary upbeat greeting to Ze is, "Hi Ze. You're a Zebra deebra, a horsy-doggy and a donkey-wonkey." She likes the sound of that so much that her eyes take on a merry glow.

—Chapter Seven—

Coco

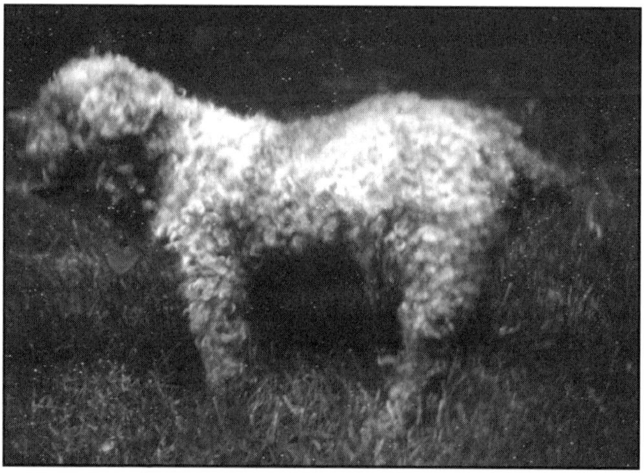

Coco was a spunky miniature brown poodle puppy that Marilyn's sister Gail adopted in 1964 from The North Shore Animal League in Port Washington, New York. We acquired her in 1984 because Gail was unable to care for her at the time.

Coco had been all alone and much enjoyed the comradeship of our dogs. She liked to bark at Bigboy, who, of course, didn't take it seriously. Coco loved to take haircuts, as evidenced every time by a visible increase in her vanity. She especially appreciated the fare at our place as opposed to the ordinary dog food she had been fed before. Her favorite treat was cheese, and she came to the breakfast table for it every morning.

As the end drew near, she became unable to climb the two steps to our back door. Staring at me, her eyes clouded, and she quietly died in her wicker basket at the grand old age of twenty-four.

Her body was buried in our backyard.

—CHAPTER EIGHT—

Casey of Dr. Suess Dals

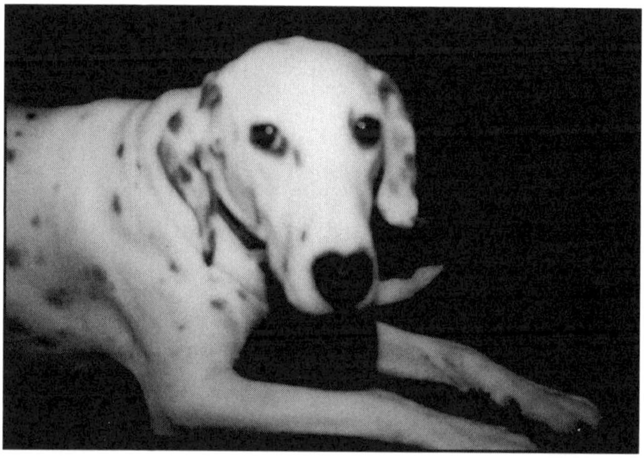

Casey was born on November 16, 1984. As sadly happens to too many Dalmatians, he wound up with the wrong person and was totally misunderstood. Above all, Dalmatians are playful and overactive. They are harlequins, and their harlequin markings are consistent with their ways. Dalmatians aim to please but must be handled firmly. Our approval is essential to them. They sometimes make their owners look silly and, when they think it's unimportant, have fun doing exactly the opposite of what they're asked. No breed is capable of more love for or needs more love from their master. In some ways, many devoted Dalmatian owners deem them to be almost their equals.

About a year after Bigboy was gone, Marilyn regularly scanned the newspaper ads. She answered one for an eight-month-old male Dalmatian. In an expression of true love, the owner, Mark Fitzgerald, had put the dog up for sale. Mark's mother was unable to tolerate the dog's quirks, and he was neutered. Mark was concerned that his mother might demand that more drastic action be taken. Despite its widespread use, castration almost never solves a behavioral problem. I know of no textbook of veterinary medicine that prescribes it for this indication.

When we entered Casey's home, he was on the second floor. At first sight, as he came down the stairs, he looked like Bigboy. He then leaped fifteen feet down the room to land on a couch. After watching the dog and talking to Mark, we decided that he was for us. Casey jumped into our car, and off we went. I stopped to get him a collar and a leash while Marilyn stayed in the car with Casey, who checked over all its components and contents.

When we arrived at home, we had a cake and ice cream party for both Ducky and Coco. For the dogs whose birth dates were unknown to us, we arbitrarily assigned their birthdays to Rani's day of birth, August first. Casey joined in the festivities as though he had been a member of the family for the longest time. He was so excited that night that he could hardly fall asleep.

Casey had light brown spots that were almost invisible on his photographs. He made himself right at home. Like King, he stole my socks and handkerchiefs as I dressed, and, like Bigboy, he ran around our circular dining table at meals. As I lay in bed, Casey enjoyed walking to and fro along the length of my back and legs. He was the only dog that Ze permitted to lick her eyes and ears.

In the winter of 1988, I had peripheral awareness that all was not well with Casey. He didn't look right, was sleeping too much, didn't want to go out in the extreme cold and developed pica for Ze's droppings. On March 25, 1988, Marilyn called me at the office to tell me that Casey was having difficulty breathing. We made an emergency visit to the vet, who conducted a thorough examination, took x-rays of Casey's lungs and collected blood. He couldn't make a diagnosis on the spot but the blood count revealed leukemia.

Early the next morning, Casey was terminal. As he died, with me holding him in my arms, a blue screen appeared before us. I realized *a priori* that it was indestructible and more than that, unassailable. It projected to Casey the most gentle, protective love imaginable, and he went to it.

Casey was Marilyn's constant companion. She loved him to distraction. In Marilyn's words, "We lived for the moment with no past, no present, no future and understood all. It was a synchrony of spirit, soul and life."

After two years and eight months of bliss, Casey's body was buried in the backyard.

—Chapter Nine—

Williamsview Maxwell Ware

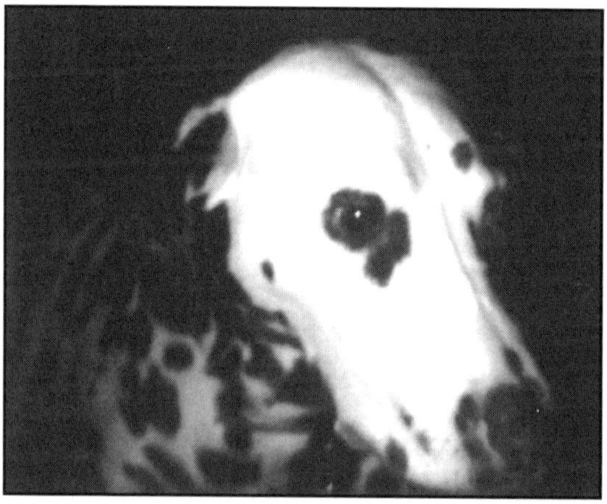

Maxwell was born on June 12, 1985, at a kennel. He too was unlucky and went to the wrong owner, one who abused him for two years before returning him to the kennel.

On a day in the winter of 1988, Marilyn missed the mail pickup and had something important to give to the postman. She set off in her car searching the neighborhood streets for the mail truck. She didn't find it but instead came to a residence in front of which a couple was walking their Dalmatian. Marilyn stopped to talk and learned that the puppy came from a kennel at which, the couple thought, other Dalmatians were for sale. Marilyn believed this was serendipity, because, with Casey gone for several months, she had been on the lookout for another Dalmatian. She contacted the kennel owner who said that the only Dal he might be willing to sell was a three-year-old male. You guessed it, it was Maxwell.

We arrived at the kennel late in the afternoon. To dazzle us, the breeder simultaneously released his many Dals from their lined-up enclosures and, all at once, they ran down their long parallel runs barking, all the way. They covered the distance in a few split seconds. It surely was an impressive sight.

When we decided to take Maxwell, the breeder exclaimed, "Not today!"

I whispered to Marilyn, "If not today, then when?"

The breeder's position seemed a paradox, because he had told us of his intention to put Maxwell down if he couldn't sell him. By this time, it had turned dark and quite cold, so we continued the conversation in his home. We were persistent and indicated that our time was valuable and that we couldn't very well keep coming back. I told him that price was no object and that we were long experienced with Dals. I think it helped that Ducky was present. After a long while, he relented and Maxwell was ours.

A few days later as I was affectionately holding Max, he began to tremble and growl. I withdrew from him carefully so as not to be mauled. This wasn't an isolated occurrence. Max went into an alternate state when we physically expressed our love for him. At bedtime, he would lie by himself, and if we walked past him, he barked so threateningly that it frightened us. We put him on a tranquilizer, which was partially effective. With time and the medication, he gradually improved. The arrival of Cheyenne, successor to Ducky, accelerated his recovery and he normalized. One can try to imagine the nature and extent of the mistreatment Max suffered in his formative years for it to have had such a profound effect on him.

While he was still manifesting his problem, Marilyn took Max with her on a visit to one of her nieces. Max was on his best behavior, but when they were back in the car about to leave, he had one of his episodes. The niece sincerely suggested that Max was telling Marilyn that he wanted to drive the car.

With all his posturing, Max never hurt either of us. He never acted out with strangers, no matter how much they admired and petted him. I guess he had to love you to go off the deep end.

Max liked to lord it over Ze, which was stressful for her. One time, he started her running and chased her. She kicked him on his head with one of her rear hooves. It made a loud popping sound, which brought to my mind a childhood memory. My father took me to a baseball game and Babe Ruth, past his prime and no longer with the Yankees, came to bat. He pointed to the stands, his characteristic gesture to let the fans know that he was going to hit a home run. The Babe no longer commanded respect, and the crowd responded with loud jeers. But when, on the next pitch, he made good on his promise, he received a standing ovation. The wild cheering went on and on. I never forgot the sound the bat made as it hit the ball, and it was the same sound Ze made when she kicked Max's head. Ze must have meant this as a warning and pulled her punch, because Max was okay. I thought he needed the lesson. Afterward, Max didn't pick on Ze again.

We had pictures of large, African cats hanging on some of our walls. Max was the only dog who ever reacted to them. He would look at them suspiciously, as though he half expected them to come out of their frames.

In 1993, routine annual laboratory tests revealed that Max was in kidney failure. At the time, renal transplants were not available for dogs. We would have taken him anywhere to have had one done. It was heartbreaking to watch such a majestic creature, our best friend, going down hill. Marilyn nursed him to the very end. Max died in uremia in May 1995.

On the sunny day before his death, Max stood facing into a brisk spring breeze for a long time. It seemed he knew he was about to leave this world and wanted to soak up for the last time one of nature's sweet bounties.

Maxwell's body was buried in our backyard.

—CHAPTER TEN—

Ravenwood Shanndal Cheyenne

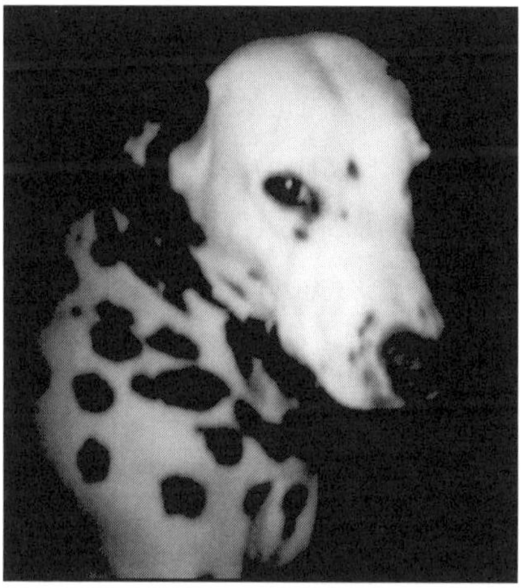

Cheyenne was born February 21, 1988 in Florida. She was acquired by a family that relocated to rural New Jersey.

In the spring of 1989, we went to see Cheyenne. At first sight, I was struck by her regal appearance. Simultaneously, she seemed to be sizing us up in her mind. We put Max and her together to see how they would react to each other. They immediately started to play-wrestle and continued doing this for twenty minutes. In fact, in the car the two of them continued their enthusiastic frolicking on the back seat all the way home.

A few days later, Marilyn noticed that the color of Cheyenne's coat was off-white between her brown spots. This discoloration didn't wash away. Cheyenne had been allowed to roam on an acreage of her former owners, and I suspect that the water on the property contaminated by some chemical. Within a year, her coat became bone white, as it should have been.

Cheyenne passed her veterinary examination with flying colors except that, for no apparent reason, her white blood count was elevated. However, the white blood count did not become normal during her entire life.

Cheyenne and Max got along famously. Only outdoors did they wrestle continually. Cheyenne would make mock surprise attacks on Max by pouncing on him at full run when he least expected it. Max became very possessive of Cheyenne and Cheyenne extremely deferential of Max.

Cheyenne had a wonderful personality. She was affectionate and easygoing. Not once did she cause trouble or create a problem. Cheyenne had a delightful sense of humor, which was expressed by her clowning manner. When we returned home from somewhere, the first thing I did was to take her for a walk along the perimeter of the property in front of our house, and she always looked forward to it.

The first indication that we had that Cheyenne's heath was failing was in December 1995 at a New Jersey State Vehicle Inspection Station. While we were waiting at the exit, she came close to collapsing, and I had to lift her back into the car. Cheyenne seemed all right until a week later when she had a visual aberration at an auto repair shop. There was a large, inlaid design on the floor, which probably looked like a puddle of water to her, because, after peering at it for a while, she carefully avoided stepping on it. The common denominator responsible for the two syndromes was auto exhaust fumes in the air in both places. Subsequently, we kept her away from fumes, and she had no further untoward reactions.

At frequent intervals in 1986, Cheyenne began having difficulty in breathing at home. The dyspnea occurred at rest and lasted several minutes. Then she developed diabetes mellitus, which required treatment with insulin. In dogs, diabetes almost never responds to oral medication. At first, I muzzled her when I administered the injections twice a day. After a time, she acceded to the injections like a good soldier, and the muzzle wasn't needed. Cheyenne once had a hypoglycemic reaction to the insulin. I inserted sugar tablets into her throat, which increased her blood glucose and reversed the reaction quickly.

On September 5, 1997, Cheyenne began to gasp for breath and froth at the mouth. I embraced her and prayed. As she slowly expired, her feeling tone was unmistakably suffused with pure love.

Cheyenne's body was buried next to Max's in the backyard.

—CHAPTER ELEVEN—

Ch Planetts Erins Acorn Jazzman

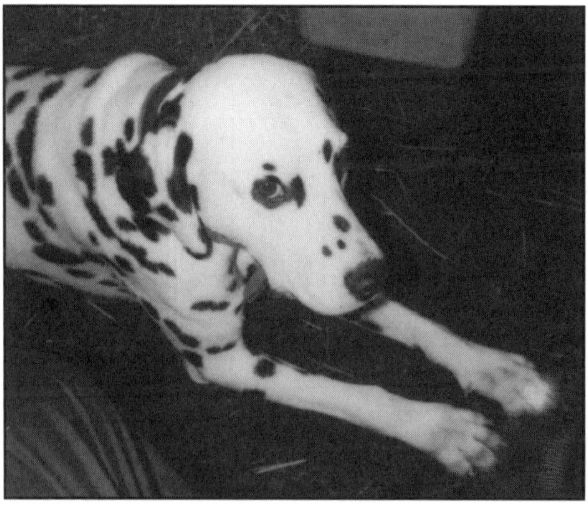

Jazz was born on March 31, 1993, and came to live with me on August 7, 1999, at the age of six-and-a-half years.

After Cheyenne's death, I became despondent and didn't seek another Dalmatian for close to two years. On August 1, 1999, I came across an intriguing newspaper ad and called the breeder, Dr. Edward Barrett, who told me that Jazz was a champion show dog — a stud — and that he was a very clean dog. He said that he would sell Jazz only on the condition that he first be neutered, because he didn't want to create competition for his business. Dr. Barrett emphasized that this condition was nonnegotiable. I replied that everything was negotiable, and we left it at that.

Marilyn once said that, in her opinion, castration impaired a dog's immune system. I pondered this roadblock to my being able to have Jazz and came up with a thought. If Jazz had a vasectomy, he would be unable to procreate, which would satisfy Dr. Barrett's condition, and he would not be altered, which would satisfy my requirement. On calling a few vets, to my surprise, I found that none of them performed that surgical procedure. A surgeon who accepted patients only on a referral basis from other vets could and would do the vasectomy.

When I presented the idea to Dr. Barrett on the phone, he accepted this solution. On my visit to see Jazz, I met the doctor, his charming wife and co-breeder, Barbara Kaplan Barrett, and their fetching daughter, Allison. I was thoroughly questioned by the Barretts, who obviously wanted to make as sure as possible that Jazz would go to a home where he would thrive and be happy. Jazz is a large, handsome Dalmatian with superb configuration. He had excoriations and abrasions on his muzzle that were believed to have happened as he climbed a tall fence. As it turned out, the Barretts were convinced that Jazz wouldn't be used as a stud and didn't require the vasectomy.

Dr. Barrett almost shed a tear as Jazz was leaving. I was supplied with some of his regular fare and an animal carrier. Dr. Barrett had to lift Jazz into my jeep, and I discovered afterwards that, to take him anywhere, I also had to lift him into the vehicle. On the ride home, Jazz lay on the floor just behind and between the front seats.

Jazz is a mindful dog who hardly ever barks. He spends his days in spirited activities, pleasant pastimes and pensive moods. His eyes are soulful, and he is the perfect example of a dignified animal.

Jazz is the most careful dog I ever knew. When he first saw Ze, he was extremely cautious and kept his distance. In a few days, he ventured closer and then realized she was no threat to him.

When I put on my socks and shoes, instead of stealing them, as King and Casey did, Jazz always leans up with his paws on my thighs and then pins me to the back of the chair with his paws on my chest. Jazz never does any of this as I *remove* my shoes and socks, however.

When I take him to a public place, Jazz invariably becomes the center of attraction. Almost everyone wants to pet him and he lets them all. Once, Jazz and I were entering the mall, two young ladies were walking behind us. One said loudly to the other, "I didn't know they let dogs in the mall."

I turned around and said, "He isn't a dog, he's a Dalmatian."

They laughed and said, "He's beautiful."

Jazz and I watched a home video in which Ducky was filmed lying in a corner of our bedroom on a crib mattress that was her bed. It hadn't been there for years. That night, when we went into the bedroom, for the first time Jazz lay down in the very spot on the floor where Ducky's bed used to be. I was flabbergasted at Jazz's power of perception and secured a crib mattress for him and positioned it in the same place as Ducky's.

In the first winter, Jazz became extremely ill. He started to bite off his tail, and, before he stopped, he shortened it by almost half. The vet said Jazz's condition was allergic, but I thought that he had a viral infection and refused treatment for hypersensitivity.

One night Jazz had difficulty breathing and came on my lap for help. The dyspnea worsened, and I remembered that one of the times Sybil was in trouble in the middle of the summer, the temperature suddenly dropped and she derived immediate benefit. I put Jazz outside, where exposure to the cold was salutary, and restored his normal respiration. Jazz gradually recovered. His running speed is up to snuff, but he sleeps a lot.

In the summer of 2000, Jazz's urine stream became diminished. Before long, even prolonged straining would pathetically produce only drops of urine. His diet was the same as that of our former Dalmatians. They were fed meat but not those high in purines. Jazz was different and formed urate stones with any kind of meat. High doses of sodium bicarbonate failed to dissolve the stones. Also, I tried placing him on allopurinol to prevent the formation of uric acid, but he was so sick he couldn't tolerate the medication.

Jazz let me catheterize him, but there was a point through which various sizes of catheters wouldn't pass. Soon, his urine flow stopped completely, and he needed emergency surgery. I took him to the hospital of Dr. Thomas Scavelli, the specialist whom I had previously contacted regarding the vasectomy. The doctor on duty that night managed to catheterize Jazz and empty his greatly distended bladder — but only after administering Valium by injection to induce relaxation.

The next day, Dr. Scavelli called from the operating room and said that he thought he would have to perform a posterior urethrostomy, the procedure that was performed on Bigboy. I earnestly asked him to just remove the stones, and he said that might not be possible if they were jammed too tightly in the urethra, the passageway within the penis. In dogs, the urethra is surrounded on three sides by bone. Fortunately, the skilled surgeon was able to evacuate all of the calculi. He reported that there were close to a hundred of them.

Postoperatively, a primary care vet branded Jazz a "stone former" and pronounced that he was doomed to repeated episodes. I placed Jazz on a meatless diet and essentially became a vegetarian myself. With some culinary knowhow, it's amazing how satisfying such a diet can be. Vegetables with high contents of purine proteins such as beans, lentils, peas and cauliflower are avoided. Mushrooms, asparagus and spinach are double threats because they contain both purines and oxalates. Certain herbs, particularly those from the parsley family, are prohibited because of their extremely high oxalate concentrations.

Jazz is all muscle and, at eighty pounds, rivals Bigboy in size and strength. We have developed a special camaraderie, and he has become my alter ego. Whether he understands me better or I him is moot.

After a run in the yard in November 2001, Jazz was unable to bear weight on his front right extremity. Naturally, I thought he had suffered an injury but examination didn't reveal evidence of this. After limping for about a week, Jazz's small toe became red and swollen. It appeared to be a bad infection, and I administered antibiotics. There was no improvement, and we consulted his doctor. X-rays disclosed a malignancy of the proximal phalanx of the toe. The next day, the toe was amputated. However, the web between the fourth and fifth toes was involved and the pathology report described an invasive osteosarcoma with a margin that was not clear (meaning that the malignant cells extended right up to an edge of the slide).

In dogs, osteosarcoma is the most common primary bone tumor and, even after prompt surgery, is considered uniformly fatal. In a follow-up procedure, Dr. Christopher Thatcher, an orthopedic surgeon at the Red Bank Veterinary Hospital in New Jersey, removed Jazz's fourth toe and portions of his fifth and fourth metacarpal bones.

To preserve Jazz's quality of life, I declined chemotherapy, which might extend survival time but is not curative. Also, I couldn't see giving Jazz a known carcinogen in the presence of a malignancy.

In March of 2002, Jazz again had difficulty urinating. He could only produce drops and repeated catheterizations weren't working. His surgeon, Dr. Benn W. Doyle of Westfield Veterinary Group, removed hundreds of urate stones from his bladder and penis.

The low-purine diet didn't work, after all. A meatless diet causes the urine to have a neutral pH, which makes administering sodium bicarbonate counterproductive because it makes the urine alkaline and promotes struvite stone formation. Now Jazz continues on his low-purine diet but, in addition, receives allopurinol to block the formation of uric acid and also to prevent de novo purine synthesis. Apparently, he was making too many of his own purines. My fingers are crossed.

—Chapter Twelve—

Erin N' Wlwd Planettstellaluna

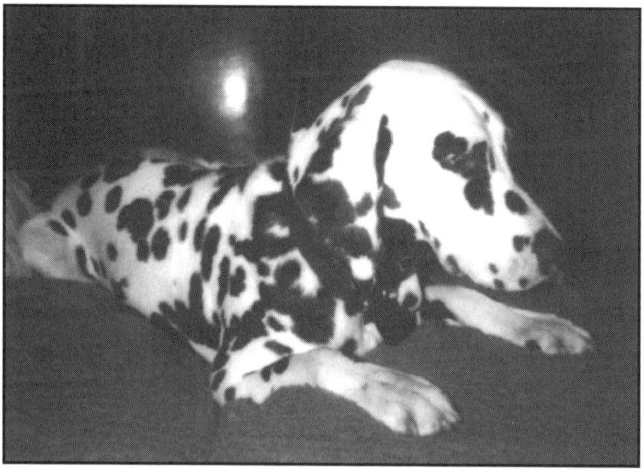

In the summer of 2000, I thought that Jazz would benefit from the companionship of a female Dalmatian. The Barretts had one for sale. She was born on October 21, 1998, and her name was Stella. On August 19, 2000, during our visit to meet Stella, Jazz tried several times to mount her. Since she was not in heat, I commented that this was unusual behavior.

The Barretts said that one of their males had been doing the same. Jazz was continuously aroused from the moment we arrived home through the entire next day. Although Stella was not receptive, he hounded her to their points of exhaustion.

Realizing that something was very wrong, I made arrangements for an emergency spaying. In addition to the routine pre-op lab tests, Dr. David Frantz ordered a blood estrogen level. The surgeon, Dr. Gregory Veronin, said that Stella's ovaries appeared normal. Her postoperative course was uneventful. The blood estrogen level turned out to be markedly elevated, exceeding the range for a dog in heat. If not corrected by removing the ovaries, hyperestrogenism is uniformly fatal in dogs. Estrogen is toxic to the bone marrow, and the animal dies from depletion of blood cells essential to life.

Stella's blood count showed that her marrow was already being affected. She was slightly anemic and her platelets were borderline low. Hopefully, the operation was performed early enough to avert Stella's premature death. Time will tell. Coming to live with Jazz may have saved Stella's life. Unless a female dog with this condition is exposed to an unaltered male, there would be no way of knowing that anything is going on until it is too late. As far as I know, there is no similar disease in the human female.

Stella is of medium size, and her body is adorned with a plethora of dark brown spots. Her ears are oversized, and she can rotate them so that their outer surfaces face forward and further beautify her quaint face. Stella's coat is unusually thick, and the end of her extra long tail looks like a fuzzy-tipped artist's brush. When Stella is preoccupied with something, she talks to herself with a repertoire of musical sounds.

Stella is irrepressibly enthusiastic. In the beginning, she would pull on her leash, run out of the house if the front door was ajar, step down hard on my bare toes, steal whatever took her fancy, chew on shoes and jump up on people. Because she is eager to learn and craves approval, she has forsaken such undisciplined inclinations in response to my disapproval of them.

Naturally, Stella likes to hunt the critters behind the house. She chases rabbits, raccoons and squirrels but so far hasn't caught one. I saw her jump six feet into the air trying to snatch a bird — and she almost did. Stella loves to climb, and when we go into the garage to collect feed for Ze, she manages to get close to the ceiling on top of the stacked bales of hay.

Stella and Jazz get along famously and show a healthy amount of competitiveness. In some ways, Stella emulates Jazz, but she is deferential and careful not to rub him the wrong way. The stud that he is, Jazz sniffs her to check every so often whether she's coming into heat. Sometimes, Jazz observes Stella intently, and, from the expression on his face, I think he considers her somewhat of a curiosity. For sure, Jazz plays the role of a kind uncle.

On Saturday March 24, 2001, Stella began to limp on her right front leg. Since she had nothing wrong with her paw, I thought that she had injured her limb or shoulder and applied traction to the extremity, to no avail. The next morning, her right front leg and tail were paralyzed. Also, she had extreme weakness in her other legs and was unable to change her position. Her breathing was labored. A dog with a sadder look never existed.

My diagnosis was polyradiculoneuritis, which is known as coon paralysis because it often follows a raccoon bite or scratch. Both the spinal cord nerve roots and peripheral nerves are affected. There is no known cause but a virus is likely. There is no curative treatment available. Spontaneous remission commonly starts within three weeks and recovery often occurs in about three months. In severe cases, this rapidly progressive neurologic illness can be fatal. In desperation, I remembered Marilyn's pronouncement that spaying or neutering an animal impairs its immune system. On Sunday, I decided to administer high doses of estrogen to Stella. It was a reach, but a miracle occurred. In twenty-four hours, slight improvement was evident. On Tuesday, Stella was able to hobble around, and, by Wednesday, her gait was normal and she could climb stairs. As always, Marilyn was right-on.

For those of you who are technically oriented and wondering what the mechanism of action of estrogen is, here goes: Estrogens activate cell nucleus receptors in the tissues of the reproductive tract and breasts, of course, but also those in the pituitary gland, the hypothalamus in the brain, the liver and bone. The activated receptors bind to certain DNA sequences, which enhance the transcription of specific adjacent genes and induce the synthesis of RNA.

—CHAPTER THIRTEEN—

Others

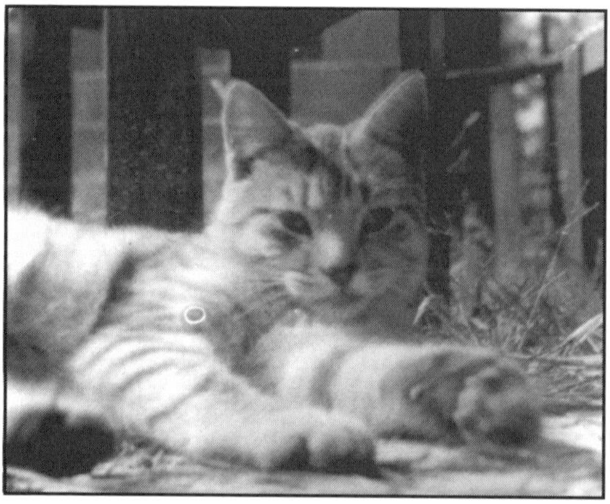

Henry was a large gray homeless cat that, at one time, probably belonged to a family that lived in the duplex rental house that we occupied in 1954 during my service at the Patuxent River Naval Air Station, which is about seventy miles Southeast of Washington, DC. Every afternoon, Henry came to the back porch for his dinner. I liked Henry and once put a collar and leash on him and took him inside. For a while, he struggled violently to free himself and then suddenly gave up and lay down. Since he didn't want to be a house cat, I returned him to the outdoors. Months later, the woman in the other duplex unit complained that Henry had jumped on her back as she hung out her wash to dry. To avoid a lawsuit, I trapped Henry, drove him miles away and set him free. I immediately had second thoughts and called to him but he was distrustful and continued to walk slowly away. I regret what I did to Henry to this day for it was morally wrong.

The first night that he was gone, I heard crying outside the house. I investigated and found a pure-white cat that must have been Henry's lover. The white female wailed every night for an entire week. This caused me to experience much guilt and sorrow. Not long after, I unexpectedly received orders to join a destroyer squadron on distant duty in the far East. The warships were performing exercises while on a round-the-world cruise. Marilyn and I didn't see each other for three months. Maybe our separation was retribution for what I did to Henry.

In the late nineteen-fifties, we were on vacation, playing golf in the Adirondack mountains when we caught sight of a thrush chick on the ground. It had fallen from its nest and was too young to fly. Next we saw an animal stalking the bird with the intention, we feared, of making a meal of it. I rescued the bird from what we believed would be a horrible death and took it back to our motel, where we fed it by dropper. On our ride home in our convertible with the top down, I placed it in the large dashboard ashtray. It made angry chirps to protest its accommodations.

Sport, as we called it, was an adorable foundling and thrived. Once it flew into a mirror in our home — probably hurting its beak, neck and pride. Generally, we didn't find it necessary to restrain Sport. It learned to fly on the beach. One day, about two months later, while driving through a wooded area, Sport jumped on the steering wheel, pecked on it three times and flew away never to be seen by us again. The call of the wild is one of the most powerful forces of nature.

In the early nineteen-sixties in New York City, we purchased two small chameleons at the circus. Actually, they were anoles, which are American lizards that can change color. We named the larger one Leon and the smaller one Camille. As time went by, our lizard family grew to five. Reptiles are devoted pets. No matter how late it was when I awakened from sleep, the lizards would remain motionless, waiting for me on a bunch of dried silver-dollar flowers that were in a vase on top of a low bookcase. When I approached, they would jump on my hands and arms.

We fed them mealworms that were stored in the refrigerator. When the mealworms were placed on the flat, perforated surface on the top of a large lamp shade, the heat from the bulb would revive them to activity, and the lizards would catch and eat them. After turning circles several times, Leon usually slept on the lower shelf of a living room cart. When we had fresh roses, he would sleep on their petals.

As I customarily did before we went out on summer days, I placed the lizards on the inside of a window screen, so that they could enjoy the weather, and then I closed the window to conserve our air conditioning. This time, when we returned, all the lizards were dead, each still clinging to the screen. Their deaths resulted from an unscheduled spraying of insecticide by the city. We were inconsolable and didn't replace the lizards.

The mid-nineteen-sixties in Norman, Oklahoma:

An older neighborhood Dalmatian named Domino would occasionally visit King. They liked each other. Domino sometimes had a large bone in his mouth. One day, we were very sad to learn that Domino's master had put him down for not staying in his yard.

Our next door neighbor's dog, Toodles, would, on her own, join King and Sybil when we went for rides to local destinations.

We had pet turtles and fish. It was a matter of concern that the tropical fish were fighting with one another. The problem was solved when we saw the famous film, "The Graduate," in which a fish tank containing three kinds of tropical fish was featured. We placed these three kinds in a tank, and they all got along peacefully. I particularly enjoyed watching the large goldfish in our cold-water tank and the plecostomus in our tropical tank. Just before we moved to Washington State, we put the cold-water fish and the turtles in a lake in the countryside. I'll never forget that one of the turtles swam back to us. This unusual show of affection was heart-warming. When the turtle was put in the lake for the second time, it didn't return.

In 1979 in New Jersey, we began putting out bird-seed. Soon thereafter, a flock of about fifty pigeons arrived. Every day and all day, they would stay behind the house on the ground and in the trees. They always departed at dusk and returned the next morning. A bird of prey almost killed a pigeon in flight, but the pigeon made a sharp turn into Ze's stable and saved itself. In February of 1983, after spending six months in Oklahoma, we came back to our home thinking that the pigeons were gone; however, one pigeon was present. It was a lookout for the flock, because the next morning, there they all were.

The last time I ever saw any of them was on December 12, 1995, on the very date that Marilyn died of a heart attack. This was a remarkable, uncanny coincidence. A few days before, Marilyn had said to me, "I will never leave you." I have no doubt that she is with me and always will be.

Epilog

Living among animals for four continuous decades and interacting with them every day has understandably modified my viewpoints.

As I see it, all animals are undeniably sentient beings and most of them are capable of reflective thought. They experience and express a spectrum of feelings. Dogs particularly have a sense of humor. They clown around not only with each other but also with persons who have developed a rapport with them. Dogs communicate with us in direct proportion to our receptivity.

The distinctive mental abilities of animals are denied or largely ignored by most of us because it enables us to put so many of them to death for food and/or to wear their body parts while maintaining a clear conscience. All of the other species have as much right to their lives as humankind does. Since animals are defenseless against us and more than ever at our mercy, we have the moral responsibility to become more benevolent toward the furry, feathered, scaly and hard-shelled denizens on the earth.

For the most part, humans either doubt that or wonder if animals go to heaven. I am convinced that animals do go to heaven. I wonder how populated heaven is with people.

About the Author

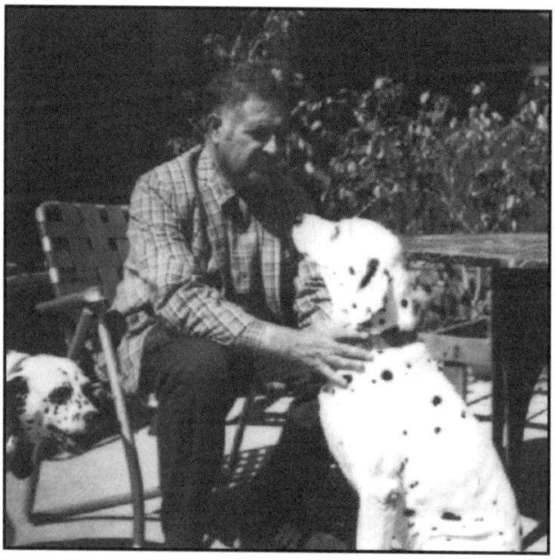

Dr. John Behrman with Big Boy and Ducky.

John Behrman graduated from the Chicago Medical School with a doctorate in medicine. He is board certified in Occupational Medicine. He has not only served in the US Naval Reserve on active duty for two years, he has been active in private practice as well as a vice president and medical director of Whitehall Laboratories, New York. Meanwhile, in his role as a physician specializing in Occupational Medicine, he has been associated with Exxon Corporation and Merck & Company.

A member of the American Medical Association and a Fellow of the American College of Preventive Medicine, he is the author of a number of published papers in his speciality.

Currently, Dr. Behrman lives and writes in Scotch Plains, New Jersey.